AMERICAN INSTITUTION

The Breakdown of the American Health Care System

Ron Burk

Table of Contents

Chapter 1 - An Unnecessary Evil

Mom had been up all night worried about a home we had just bought and in her delirium, she forgot whether she gave my little brother Keith his Prednisone, a shot-in-the-dark derivative of Cortisone he was prescribed to treat Rheumatoid Arthritis. Or at least that's what the doctors thought he had after years of pricking him with needles and performing countless tests trying to diagnose the endless flu he developed after taking a routine flu shot when he was a healthy, happy four-year-old. He had spent years in the hospital, including one agonizing 18-month stint in Children's Hospital near Los Angeles.

Worried sick that he might get worse, Mom chose to rush him back to Children's. I remember thinking he would be fine. He had started walking again and wore a back brace from the years of crippling hospitalization. That's what the Prednisone was for, to give him relief from the back pain that developed from all those years in the hospital.

When I visited him days later, he had gotten much worse and was now in an oxygen tent. Still, I was sure he would recover. His happy nature had returned when he came home from the years-long hospital stay and he had been excited to start second grade, as broken as his body had become.

Two weeks passed and I had just enrolled in my freshman year of high school when Mom and Dad came home in the middle of the night. 'Keith's dead!' she cried out, sobbing uncontrollably. I was in shock! He was getting better at home. How could this happen? Mom was never the same after that, a perpetual veil of sadness shadowed her every movement, and shrieks of guilt and despair came from their bedroom every night for years after that as she woke to realize what had happened. She blamed herself and, in a way, she was right. It was my first encounter with the devastation caused by long-term stays at that bastion of hope, the American Institution, I.e., the hospital.

Many years passed and our family was destroyed, Mom perpetually reliving the nightmare of that night. It was years before Dad revealed to me the words Keith said to him from inside that oxygen tent, words that would become all too clear when I found myself hospitalized for several weeks some 55 years later...

"Daddy," he said to my father. "I want to die."

Chapter 2 – A Perfect Storm

Life was almost perfect. I was 67 and looked 20 years younger than my years. I had never been sick a day in my life and I had the physique of a young man. I felt as though I would never age. I married the girl of my dreams. She was and is the most beautiful girl I have ever seen... a vision not unlike that of Marilyn Monroe. She also shared the gift of youth. All the men wanted her, and still do. I was the lucky man to marry her. We had bought a home in the beautiful Angeles National Forest in Southern California located in an idyllic little slice of heaven 60 miles north of Los Angeles called Green Valley. There were only two stores in the whole town, and everyone knew you by your first name. I always wondered if these 200-year-old oak trees could talk, what would they say? It was God's country.

But not all was perfect in LaLa land. My auto advertising business, after 30 years of success, was nearly shut down in the wake of the Covid scare. Detroit had made a near fatal error. While building their cars with American hands and machines, the brains powering today's modern marvels were tiny swatches of silicon built in another country and had become unattainable in the days of Covid 19. New cars were backed up in the factories and on the docks of America, lacking a wafer-sized silicon chip needed to power them up to ship to dealers and then to the American public.

No one expected it to last so long, but the crisis continued as months turned into years.

We chose to move in with my wife Christine's mom in sunny Florida, half a world away. She went ahead of me to see if such an arrangement was possible. And if it was, I would ship the dogs and sell the house. But there was more to the story than even I knew. Christine was upset at me for failing her so miserably and considered divorce. That's when all hell broke loose. It had been a year since my main client had hired me. New car sales had dropped to almost zero and what is the good of advertising to sell something you can't order in stock to sell?

So now I was driving for Door Dash, not a horrible gig, but at the end of the day, you eke out a minimal living after gas, and surely not enough to support my wife, myself, utilities, our half-dozen dogs and cover the inevitable problems that arise when you use your car to deliver food all day. Potholes took out two wheels and tires in a single month.

On the home front, a storm came through and dropped nine trees on our property including one oak that was so large it filled the front yard, blocking access completely. Just a few days later, eighteen inches of snow fell. When I could show the house, the dogs went wild, and our big crazy German Shepherd bit a prospective buyer. I was at the end of the rope and my stress level went through the roof.

It was another beautiful day in what should have been paradise, and I stepped outside of the house and as I walked down the sidewalk, my body began to freeze up. I was having a stroke from the stress. Somehow, I was able to drive my car to one of the two local stores, where they called the ambulance.

Chapter 3 - Mad Science

I always had a fear of hospitals after my brother's death. As the years went by, I found out that no one dies from the supposed disease that gripped my little brother. And as the years passed, I discovered that the autopsy showed there were over 200 needle marks in his fragile little body, the result of doctors using him as an experimental science project, not knowing what to do except to stab and poke and test and test some more. I never forgot his desperate call for help, "Daddy, I want to die!"

The ambulance dropped me in the halls of the emergency room where I waited four hours for a room. The ambulance crew stayed with me and informed the nurses that I'd had a stroke. A shot right then and there of Antiplatelet would have cleared the arteries going to my brain and would have saved me months of paralysis.

There is a well-known period when a stroke occurs called "the golden hour." The golden hour in the context of a medical emergency refers to a critical period following a traumatic injury or the onset of certain medical conditions, particularly a stroke. During this time, rapid medical intervention can significantly improve a patient's chances of survival and recovery.

For strokes, the golden hour typically refers to the first 60 minutes after the onset of symptoms. Strokes can be ischemic (caused by a blocked blood vessel in the brain) or hemorrhagic (caused by bleeding in the brain). In either case, prompt medical attention is crucial.

Here's why the golden hour is important for stroke care:

Tissue Salvage: In ischemic strokes, brain tissue begins to die when it doesn't receive an adequate blood supply. Rapid treatment, such as administering a clot-busting medication like tissue plasminogen activator (tPA) or performing a thrombectomy, can restore blood flow and prevent further damage to the brain.

Minimizing Disability: Quick treatment can also minimize the extent of disability following a stroke. The longer it takes to receive treatment, the greater the risk of permanent brain damage and long-term impairment.

Recovery and Rehabilitation: Early intervention allows for a faster start to the recovery and rehabilitation process. Stroke patients who receive prompt care are more likely to regain lost functions and independence.

Recognizing the signs of stroke and acting swiftly is essential. Common stroke symptoms include:

Numbness or weakness in the face, arm, or leg, especially on one side of the body.

Trouble speaking or understanding speech.

Confusion, trouble with vision, or difficulty walking.

Severe headache with no known cause.

If you or someone you are with experiences these symptoms, it's important to call emergency services immediately. The faster medical attention is received, the better the chances of a positive outcome. In the case of a stroke, time truly is of the essence, and the golden hour can make a life-changing difference.

In my case, not only did the hospital fail to give me a life-changing blood thinner, but they also deprived me of food, water and medical treatment for four full days! They checked my blood, did a urinalysis and two mind-jarring cat scans, but performed no medical treatment. Why should they? The first thing they had me do was sign away my rights to sue them for something they failed to do. As long as they did nothing, they were in the clear.

When you sign a hospital admittance form, you are granting the hospital permission to provide you with medical care and treatment, and you are agreeing to abide by the hospital's rules and policies while you are under their care. Here are some important points to consider:

Medical Treatment: By signing the admittance form, you are giving consent for the hospital's medical staff to evaluate, diagnose, and treat your medical condition. You have the right to be informed about the proposed treatment and to make decisions about your care, including the right to refuse treatment (in most cases).

Privacy: You still have the right to medical privacy under laws like the Health Insurance Portability and Accountability Act (HIPAA) in the United States. Your medical information should be kept confidential, and you have the right to access your medical records.

Informed Consent: Before any significant medical procedure, you should be informed of the risks, benefits, and alternatives, and you have the right to provide informed consent or refuse treatment based on that information.

Refusal of Treatment: You can refuse any treatment, including life-saving treatment, as long as you are deemed competent to make that decision. However, the medical staff may seek a second opinion or consult with an ethics committee if they believe your decision may be harmful to your well-being.

Personal Property: While you are in the hospital, you may be asked to store your personal belongings or valuables. You should receive an inventory of items, and the hospital is generally responsible for safeguarding your property.

Visitation Rights: You have the right to receive visitors in accordance with the hospital's visitation policy, unless there are medical or safety reasons that limit or restrict visitation.

Discharge: You cannot be discharged from the hospital without your consent unless you are deemed medically stable and safe to leave, or if you are a danger to yourself or others. You should receive written notice of your discharge rights.

Complaints and Grievances: You have the right to voice complaints or grievances about your care without fear of retaliation. Hospitals often have a formal process for addressing patient concerns.

It's essential to read and understand any forms you are asked to sign when you are admitted to a hospital. If you have questions or concerns about your rights or the content of the forms, you can seek clarification from the hospital staff or, if necessary, consult with a patient advocate or legal counsel. Your rights as a patient are generally protected by law, and hospitals have a duty to respect and uphold those rights.

However, they can also hold you against your will for three days while they evaluate you.

A psychiatric hold, also known as an involuntary psychiatric hospitalization or psychiatric commitment, is a legal process by which individuals can be involuntarily admitted to a hospital or psychiatric facility for evaluation and treatment. The specific laws and procedures for psychiatric holds vary by jurisdiction, but a single doctor can start the process. Here are some general principles:

Criteria for Involuntary Commitment: In most places, involuntary commitment is typically reserved for individuals who pose a significant risk to themselves or others due to a severe mental health condition. The criteria for involuntary commitment can include evidence of danger to self or others, severe impairment in judgment, or an inability to meet basic needs.

Emergency Commitment: In emergency situations where there is an immediate risk to the person or others, a mental health professional or law enforcement officer can initiate an emergency psychiatric hold. This allows for a brief period of observation and assessment in a hospital or psychiatric facility.

Court-Ordered Commitment: For longer-term involuntary commitment, a court process is usually involved. A mental health professional, family member, or concerned party may file a petition with the court to request involuntary commitment. The court then conducts a hearing to determine if the individual meets the criteria for commitment.

Duration of Commitment: The length of an involuntary commitment can vary widely depending on the jurisdiction and the individual's condition. It can range from a few days to several weeks or even longer in some cases. Periodic reviews may be conducted to assess whether continued hospitalization is necessary.

Rights of the Individual: Individuals who are subject to involuntary psychiatric holds still have certain legal rights. These rights can include the right to legal representation, the right to challenge the commitment in court, and the right to receive appropriate treatment in the least restrictive setting possible.

Treatment and Evaluation: While under psychiatric hold, individuals receive psychiatric assessment and treatment to stabilize their condition. The goal is to provide the necessary care to address their mental health issues and minimize the risk to themselves and others.

Release: Individuals who no longer meet the criteria for involuntary commitment may be released from the hospital or psychiatric facility. Depending on the situation, they may be referred to outpatient care, therapy, or other community-based mental health services.

It's important to note that the procedures and laws surrounding psychiatric holds can vary significantly from one jurisdiction to another. Additionally, safeguards are often in place to ensure that individuals are not subject to involuntary commitment arbitrarily and that their rights are protected throughout the process. If you or someone you know is facing involuntary commitment, it is advisable to consult with an attorney or advocate who is familiar with mental health law in your area to understand your rights and options.

Because the hospital failed to treat me with a blood thinner in that first hour, left-side paralysis set in and while not permanent, it has required thousands of hours of therapy and kept me from working for months, exasperating my original stress tremendously. I must admit, I hated what I had become and was massively insecure about my chances of ever being more than "half a man" again with my beautiful wife. I hated the hospital until I realized I had to release it for Christine and me to ever have a chance in the future.

Long-term hospitalization, while sometimes necessary for serious medical conditions, can pose several dangers and challenges to patients. These dangers include:

Muscle Atrophy: Extended bed rest can lead to muscle weakness and atrophy, making it difficult for patients to regain their strength and mobility.

Pressure Ulcers: Immobility can result in pressure sores, which are painful and can lead to serious infections if not managed properly.

Infections: Hospital-acquired infections are a concern, especially for patients with weakened immune systems due to prolonged stays.

Depression and Anxiety: Long-term hospitalization can lead to feelings of isolation, helplessness, and depression. The sterile hospital environment and lack of social interaction can contribute to these issues.

Cognitive Decline: Some patients may experience cognitive decline or confusion due to the stress and confinement of a hospital setting.

Loss of Skills: Extended stays may lead to a loss of basic life skills, such as self-care and activities of daily living.

Dependence on Caregivers: Patients may become overly dependent on healthcare providers, making it challenging for them to regain independence once they leave the hospital.

Medical Costs: Long-term hospitalization can result in substantial medical bills, even with insurance coverage.

Lost Income: Patients and their families may experience financial strain due to lost wages and the cost of hospitalization.

Limited Social Interaction: Long-term hospitalization can result in social isolation, which can be detrimental to a patient's emotional well-being.

Strained Relationships: Family and friend relationships can become strained due to the prolonged absence and the emotional toll of caregiving.

Exposure to Disease: Prolonged stays in hospitals increase the exposure to various pathogens, which can increase the risk of hospital-acquired infections.

Medication Risks: Long-term use of medications may lead to side effects or complications, and patients may become dependent on certain medications.

Quality of Life: Prolonged hospitalization can negatively impact a patient's overall quality of life, including their ability to participate in activities they enjoy.

Stigmatization and Psychological Impact: Some patients may feel stigmatized by their extended hospital stay, which can affect their self-esteem and self-worth.

It's important to note that while long-term hospitalization carries these risks, it is sometimes the best or only option for patients with severe or complex medical conditions. Healthcare providers work to minimize these risks through various interventions, such as physical therapy, psychological support, and infection control measures. Additionally, home care and rehabilitation programs may be options to facilitate a patient's transition back to a more normal life when appropriate.

Rehabilitation of my paralysis was made much more difficult by the back pain that set in due to the long hospital stay. When I even tried to sit up, an alarm would sound, and I would be told to lay back down.

The hospital's fear of being sued extended to stopping the mere act of sitting up.

Back pain is a common issue that can develop as a result of long hospital stays. Several factors contribute to this problem:

Prolonged Bed Rest: Patients in long-term hospitalization often spend extended periods in bed, which can lead to muscle stiffness and weakness in the back. The lack of movement can cause the muscles to atrophy, and this can lead to discomfort and pain in the lower back.

Pressure Ulcers: Patients who are immobile for extended periods are at a higher risk of developing pressure ulcers or bedsores. These sores can be painful and are commonly found on the lower back, buttocks, and other bony prominences.

Poor Ergonomics: Hospital beds and chairs may not provide the best ergonomic support. Prolonged sitting or lying in positions that don't adequately support the spine can lead to back pain.

Medication Side Effects: Some medications given during hospital stays, such as opioids for pain management, can cause constipation. Straining during bowel movements due to constipation can exacerbate or trigger back pain.

Stress and Anxiety: Being in a hospital for an extended period can be stressful and anxiety-inducing, which can lead to muscle tension and exacerbate existing back pain.

Lack of Physical Activity: Physical therapy and regular mobility are essential for preventing and managing back pain. Prolonged hospitalization can limit a patient's ability to engage in physical activity, leading to deconditioning and muscle imbalances that contribute to back pain.

Inadequate Mattress or Bed: The quality of the hospital bed or mattress can play a role in back pain. An uncomfortable or unsupportive surface can lead to discomfort and spinal misalignment.

To help prevent or manage back pain during long hospital stays, healthcare providers can take several measures:

Encourage and assist patients in performing gentle mobility exercises and changing positions regularly.

Provide appropriate support surfaces like pressure-relief mattresses.

Ensure proper pain management strategies that don't rely solely on opioid medications.

Educate patients and caregivers on proper body mechanics and ergonomics.

Use cushions or pillows to support the patient's back and maintain proper alignment.

It's essential for patients to communicate any discomfort or pain they experience to their healthcare team. Managing back pain during long hospital stays is a collaborative effort between patients and healthcare providers to minimize discomfort and promote recovery.

I was one of two patients who would walk (with a cane) up and down the corridors during therapy. Another was a woman and when we would pass each other we would say "hi." By the time a month had passed, she no longer waved, instead staring blankly ahead. She had become a zombie. I knew I had to get out of there. Everyone was losing their minds, me included. The total alienation from normalcy made time almost stand still. I am reminded of the line from the Bible, "a day is as a thousand years."

Now I understood why my brother fell into despair when faced with going back to the hospital. Now I understood why he told my dad, "I want to die." It was literally turning into an insane asylum. I began to think differently, focusing on one thing only... my escape from this hell.

Precious few members of the hospital staff understood what I was going through. A few did understand, and were compassionate, but helpless to help. Most were disconnected from the patients by the grueling 12-hour days, three-on, three-off work schedules and rotation through various floors and buildings.

The compassion and empathy of hospital staff are influenced by various factors, and the number of hours worked, as well as the rotation schedule are among them. Prolonged hours and demanding rotations can potentially impact the compassionate care provided by healthcare professionals in several ways:

Compassion Fatigue: Healthcare workers who are consistently overworked or have long shifts can experience compassion fatigue. This is a state of emotional exhaustion and reduced empathy caused by the constant exposure to the suffering and pain of patients. As a result, they may become desensitized or detached, affecting their ability to provide compassionate care.

Burnout: Prolonged hours and frequent rotations can contribute to burnout, which is characterized by physical and emotional exhaustion, cynicism, and reduced effectiveness at work. Burnout can lead to decreased motivation to provide compassionate care and increased irritability.

Decreased Patient Interaction: Longer work hours and frequent rotations may leave healthcare professionals with less time and energy to spend with each patient. This reduced interaction time can make it challenging to develop strong patient-provider relationships, which are crucial for compassionate care.

Mistakes and Errors: Fatigue from long hours and frequent rotations can impair cognitive function and decision-making, potentially leading to mistakes or errors in patient care. These errors can negatively affect patient outcomes and may reduce healthcare providers' confidence in their ability to provide compassionate care.

Reduced Work-Life Balance: Healthcare professionals who work long hours and have unpredictable rotation schedules may struggle to maintain a healthy work-life balance. This imbalance can lead to increased stress and decreased overall well-being, which can, in turn, affect their ability to provide compassionate care.

Impact on Self-Care: Healthcare workers may neglect their own physical and emotional needs when working long hours or on challenging rotations. This can lead to personal health issues and hinder their ability to provide quality care.

It's important to note that not all healthcare professionals will experience a decrease in compassion or empathy due to long hours or rotations. Many are dedicated to their patients and work diligently to provide compassionate care under challenging circumstances. I had one caregiver who called me months after my release to see how I was doing.

Healthcare institutions can take steps to mitigate the negative effects of long hours and demanding rotations on compassion and empathy, including:

Implementing policies to limit excessive working hours.

Providing support programs for healthcare workers, such as counseling and stress management.

Promoting a culture of work-life balance and self-care.

Offering training in empathy and compassionate communication to healthcare staff.

Encouraging teamwork and mutual support among healthcare teams.

Ultimately, the goal is to create working conditions that allow healthcare professionals to provide the best possible care while maintaining their own well-being.

Even family members failed to realize the negative physical and psychological aspects of long-term hospitalization, believing it was the best place for me, the place where I was safe and could get "good medical care." They rested easy in their beds at night, living life somewhat normally, thinking the hospital was "the safest place for me to get the care I needed," while in reality, I was losing my mind. When looking back, I am reminded of the movie, starring Jack Nicolson, "One Flew Over the Cuckoo's Nest." But thank God for Christine. She alone believed me when I told her I was losing my mind. She saved me by approving my release against doctor's orders. I waited for my ride on the day of my release hoping and praying nothing would go wrong. I felt as if I was escaping prison.

Chapter 4 - A Taste of Hell

I know now just a small sliver of the hell my brother Keith endured. While he suffered, I was learning to swim in the pool at the local Travel Lodge motel, where we lived to be close to him during his year and a half at Children's Hospital. When they finally released him after four long years of poking, prodding and failed diagnoses, eighteen months straight confined to a hospital bed, he felt the warm sun on his face again. In pain, he struggled to walk but loved every minute free of the hell the medical system forced on him. When he was readmitted because mom forgot whether he got his pill that day or not, life on Earth ended for him. He spiraled into the only sure escape he knew. He died.

Hospital stays should generally be as short as possible for several reasons:

Cost-Effective: Hospitals are expensive, and longer stays result in higher healthcare costs. By keeping hospital stays short, healthcare systems can allocate resources more efficiently and reduce the financial burden on patients and insurance providers.

Reduced Risk of Infections: Especially with the advent of Covid-19, the longer a patient stays in a hospital, the higher the risk of acquiring a hospital-acquired infection

(HAI). Shorter stays can help minimize this risk and improve patient safety.

Emotional and Psychological Well-Being: Prolonged hospital stays can lead to emotional and psychological stress for patients. Being away from home, family, and familiar surroundings can contribute to anxiety and depression. Shorter stays can help mitigate these negative effects.

Faster Recovery: In many cases, patients recover faster when they can return to their homes and daily routines. Hospitals can be stressful environments, and being in one for an extended period may slow down the healing process.

Bed Availability: Hospitals often have limited bed capacity, and shorter stays free up beds for other patients who may need urgent care. This ensures that healthcare resources are available to those who need them most.

Rehabilitation in Home Environment: Some patients require rehabilitation or ongoing care after their hospital stay. In many cases, this can be accomplished more effectively in the patient's home or in a less intensive care setting, which promotes a more comfortable and supportive environment.

Minimized Exposure to Medical Errors: The longer a patient stays in a hospital, the greater the potential for medical errors, such as medication mistakes or misdiagnoses. Reducing the length of hospital stays can help minimize these risks.

Patient Preference: Many patients prefer to recover at home, surrounded by their loved ones and familiar surroundings. Shorter hospital stays align with patient preferences and promote patient-centered care.

However, it's important to note that the appropriate length of a hospital stay varies depending on the individual patient's condition and needs. In some cases, longer hospitalization may be necessary for complex medical conditions or surgical procedures. The goal is to strike a balance between ensuring patients receive the necessary care and minimizing the duration of their hospital stay when possible. Additionally, advances in medical technology and healthcare delivery may continue to influence the ideal length of hospital stays in the future.

Chapter 5 - Alive Again

Once I got back to my home, my condition started improving rapidly. Being free to get up out of bed and dictate my own routine was immensely helpful. My mind came back first. My friend Daniel, who helped me out while at home, informed Christine of my horrible physical condition, which scared her, but he also told her my mental condition was improving by leaps and bounds, which made her jump for joy that she had done the right thing in getting me released. I felt human again. I was improving daily.

Medicare paid to have therapists visit me every week. While it might seem expensive, it's far less expensive than taking up space in a brick-and-mortar hospital. Once coverage of that therapy ran out, one of my therapists suggested going at least once to a therapy gym and learning the routine and then working out at Planet Fitness or its equivalent, applying the knowledge I had learned. "If I told everyone to do that, I'd be out of a job!" she said. It requires some amount of discipline, but I have no problem with that.

Whether home care is better than hospital care depends on various factors, including the individual's medical condition, the level of care required, and personal preferences. Both home care and hospital care have their advantages, and the choice between the two should be made on a case-by-case basis.

The advantages of Home Care include:

Comfort and Familiarity: Being in the comfort of one's own home can provide emotional and psychological comfort, which can be important for healing and well-being.

Independence: Home care allows individuals to maintain a level of independence and control over their daily routines.

Personalized Care: Caregivers can provide one-on-one attention, which can lead to more personalized care tailored to the individual's needs.

Reduced Risk of Infections: Hospitals can expose patients to a higher risk of infections, while home care can reduce this risk.

Lower Cost: Home care can be more cost-effective compared to hospital care, especially for long-term care needs.

Disadvantages of home care include:

Limited Medical Resources: Home care may have limitations in terms of medical equipment and resources compared to hospitals.

Lack of Immediate Medical Attention: In emergency situations, access to medical professionals and specialized equipment may be slower in a home care setting.

Caregiver Availability: The availability of caregivers and their level of training can vary, potentially affecting the quality of care.

Limited Monitoring: Continuous monitoring of vital signs and medical conditions may be less robust in a home setting.

Inadequate Space: Some medical conditions require specialized facilities and equipment that may not be available at home. Don't forget though, that much of the therapy equipment is the same as what's available at your local gym. Gyms like Planet Fitness are well equipped and can run asl little as $10 per month.

Chapter 6 - Why Bad Things Happen to Good People

It's hard to figure out why "bad things happen to good people," but life improved immeasurably after the stroke. Christine and I both agree I would still be stuck in Green Valley with the dogs, which means the house would not have sold and she would have come back to what had turned into an arduous stress-filled life for us. Our marriage would possibly not have survived.

Instead, because of my stroke, neighbors rallied around us and three of them flew our dogs to Florida. Another cleaned the house so it would sell fast and now that we're here and there are so many more advertising opportunities, we can start making money again. Christine and her mother had lived apart for so long, they had developed personality clashes, they are both so head strong. But now their relationship has vastly improved. Chrissy and I play music together, with her on vocals and me on guitar. My hand is improving, and I'm determined to play guitar better than ever, plus while LA's music industry was dead, there's hundreds of places to play here in Florida. Our house sold and the future is looking brighter than ever.

It's a story that is echoed by what happened to my friend Clyde, who I thank forever for giving me a ride that day to rescue me from the hospital. Not long after my stroke, someone burned down his house and his son died in the fire.

His son had problems and Clyde worked long hours to take care of him. The boy was schizoid, and another personality had emerged, taking complete control over his body. After the fire, Clyde came to understand that God took his child and watches over him in heaven. Clyde has started a new life, free of the burden of watching his boy sink into the darkness. Clyde now teaches others about the perils of split personalities.

The question of why bad things happen to good people is a deeply philosophical and complex one, and it has been a topic of debate and discussion for centuries. There is no one-size-fits-all answer, as people's beliefs and perspectives on this issue can vary widely based on their religious, philosophical, or personal views. Here are some common explanations and perspectives:

Randomness and Probability: Some people argue that bad things can happen to anyone because the world is inherently random and unpredictable. Events like accidents, natural disasters, or illnesses are often seen because of chance and probability, rather than a reflection of a person's character or goodness.

Free Will and Moral Choices: Another perspective is that humans have free will, and their choices and actions can lead to both good and bad outcomes. This view suggests that some bad things happen because of the choices made by individuals, and it's not always a matter of cosmic justice.

Social and Environmental Factors: Some bad things that happen to people are a result of broader social, economic, or environmental factors. Inequities in access to resources, healthcare, education, and opportunities can lead to individuals facing adversity, even if they are personally virtuous.

Psychological Perspective: From a psychological standpoint, individuals' perceptions of events and their resilience in the face of adversity can vary widely. What one person may see as a "bad" thing happening to them, another person may view as a challenge to overcome and grow from.

Complex Interplay: Often, it seems a combination of various factors contribute to life's outcomes. These can include individual choices, external circumstances, and factors beyond one's control.

Theodicy and Religious Beliefs: In many religious traditions, there are explanations for suffering and adversity. For example, in Christianity, some believe that suffering is a test of faith, a means of personal growth, or a way to fulfill a larger divine plan. In other faiths, karma or reincarnation may play a role in understanding the distribution of good and bad experiences.

It's important to note that people's views on this topic can be deeply personal and may be influenced by their own experiences, beliefs, and cultural backgrounds. The question of why bad things happen to good people remains a complex and enduring philosophical question, and different people may find solace and understanding in different explanations.

But one explanation that is more ethereal is that God simply intervened. It seemed that when this flurry of events came at us, there was an invisible force at work... I now understand it was the hand of God. Sometimes it seems as though one bad thing after another happens to us and we are unable to control the outcome. In the long run, things become clear as our life changes seemingly inexplicitly for the better. An analogy Christine and I have come to believe is that sometimes you need to lose a job to gain a better one. Sometimes you are forced out of your home, and you wind up in a better place. Often people who are suffering here on Earth die to get to heaven... like my brother and Clyde's son.

Our minds don't always conceive of the greater picture. One thing is for sure, this world didn't just happen by accident, the result of a big bang out of nothingness and the unlikely evolution of a microbe growing into a human being. There is way too much design behind fate. We are the work of God.

I write this book today not as a testament to pain, but as a warning to the world that I hope will save countless lives.

Believe in getting your loved one home as quickly as possible. Understand that hospitals were made for short term healing only. The consequences of long-term hospitalization can be manifest and fatal. Long-term hospital stays are often more deadly than the disease itself. And there is no better healer than love.